BREAKING THE MOLD

Tim Taylor

ISBN: 1463678290
ISBN-13:978-1463678296

DEDICATION

This book was not even in my thought process until one day when I was checking my email and there was a comment from a long time client of mine and his comment was that he recently saw a bunch of videos on the web on how to change up his workouts so he could keep growing and stop plateauing. I had known him when I had worked at another health spa but had left so we had lost contact until that email. His comment made me laugh because the last sentence said so master trainer since you are a flowing fountain of information, what do you recommend to help me with my upper body? Now do not get me wrong Andrew in no way, shape or form is small. In fact he is what most would call a freak of nature with his bulk and overall lean muscle mass. The guy is a beast and eats like a monster all the right foods and trains more than most people I know. Trying to do a body fat analysis on him was no easy task. The only thing you were pinching was muscle and hair but no fat and so vascular it was incredible. So when I got an email from him asking for my advice I was inspired to begin writing a book about advanced body building and advanced techniques.

When you walk into most book stores you notice a ton of books dedicated to the beginner or novice but not one dedicated to people who have made this a lifestyle and just keep on plateauing because they have tried it all. On the other hand there are tons of magazines out there but the problem becomes that most are just another advertisement to sell yet another supplement. So Andrew Randolph and all of you that want that extra lean mass and bulk this book is hereby dedicated to you. Hope you enjoy it !

Tim Taylor

CONTENTS

1 BREAKING IN

This book was designed with one thing in mind and that is to break the mold and break the theory of building lean muscle, getting more shredded and larger than ever. This book was not written for the beginning or even novice weight lifter this book was written with the intention of assisting those who are serious about working out, who hit the gym on a daily basis, have maybe hit a plateau point or are in introductory competition and want the edge needed to succeed and be victorious.

This program is designed to give your muscles no other choice but to grow bigger it is just that simple. There are a bunch of programs that guarantee the same results but with the use of either steroids or other supplements. If you have been bodybuilding for a while you are not new to the supplement world and some of you may have even experimented using steroids. In this book I do not go deeply at all into supplements because the stage you are at, reading this book any supplement information you need I am sure you are aware you can get every month in every muscle magazine out there.

There is a lot of science behind bodybuilding more than most people realize. Fact is this the older we get the harder it is to build and maintain muscle mass it is just reality. Testosterone levels go down and a number of factors come into play.

Muscles are comprised into what we in the bodybuilding world refer to as individual muscle fibers. What your ultimate goal is here is to make those individual fibers become even thicker . If your fibers do not become thicker than you will not add that mass you want to your body. Since you are already an experienced bodybuilder or fitness enthusiast whichever way you want to look at it, you should already be aware of the plateau effect and changing up your workouts, sets, repetitions, range of motion, tempo and intensity. Now what I must do is design you an effective program that will force your body into having no choice but to grow bigger and bigger. If you eat correctly and follow this program there is no reason that you should not see a visible difference in muscle size in weeks.

Now if you had read my other book "THE ABC's OF A LEAN SCULPTED BODY" You will recall the triangle of fundamentals. The triangle I am referring to was for the beginner now that you are in the advanced stage of bodybuilding we need to expand on the triangle:

The basic triangle consisted of Food, Cardio, Strength Training we are now going to add three more elements to that called Intensity, Volume and Frequency.

Let us tear right into this:

Food, deprived of food we have no dynamism and it is the appropriate nourishment we are conversing about here which once again you should know by now. With food we include water. Your muscles are comprised of water and protein, if we absence them from our diet, than our muscles will not properly rebuild.

Cardio, without a good cardio program we do not get our blood circulating the correct way and do not keep our stamina where it needs to be, again basic beginner logic. However you are going to notice a huge change with cardio later in this program.

Strength Training, which was always the big one on the bottom of the triangle but will now also have other aspects added to it.

Intensity being how much soreness, perspiration, tears, and physically taxing we going to make these workouts.

Volume being the expansiveness of exercise as well as the maneuvers you will be performing.

Frequency being how often you will be working out your body.

There is more to this entire philosophy and if you hunger to maximize your increases in muscular size, it is imperative for you to comprehend and absorb some very important dynamics. Some of the aspects I want to place emphasis on are muscle fibers, evolution, and the anaerobic training window.

There is a point in an exercise set where our growth mechanism is initiated below that point however no muscular development is stimulated. You must cross this brink which I call the point of failure. When you reach the point in an exercise set where you cannot feasibly complete another positive repetition independently you can say you have reached failure.

Muscle growth is essentially a protection device by the body, which is another fact that many newcomers are not aware of. Much in the same way that a blood clot or a suntan is. Of course, a sufficient motivation is required to produce this type of adaptation .Unfortunately for us humans, our bodies would much rather we built no muscle whatsoever.

Muscle is metabolically active tissue, the more of it you have, the more calories that are required to keep you thriving. Our bodies have adapted to expect long periods of hunger. They are also very efficient at storing body fat in anticipation of these starvation periods.

Modern man is faced with the dilemma of wanting to be lean and muscular, while our body desires us to have no excess muscle beyond normal levels of course and a ready supply of fat if or when famine strikes.

Our most powerful muscle fibers, and the ones that respond most to weight training, are our type 2 fibers. These are our fast-twitch, anaerobic power fibers. There are Type 1 fibers which are slow twitch and type 2a, 2ab, and 2b fibers which are fast twitch
Here is the interesting thing about muscle fibers: They are recruited chronologically. This means that as a set escalates in intensity and muscle fibers fatigue, more fibers are recruited from the next fiber type in the following order:
Type 1
Type 2a
Type 2ab
Type 2b

It should be rational to say, if we want to recruit and fatigue our type two fibers, we have to bring our set to a point where sufficient intensity is occurring to call into play the relevant motor units for the type 2b fibers.

In everyday life our brain will not send out this indicator unless there is some sort of alternative situation at hand. However, muscle hackers can voluntarily recruit these fibers by working to a point of muscular failure.

Let us take an example a gentleman does a set of ten reps, the tenth rep being the last rep possible, he will not be involving his type 2b fibers until the 9th or 10th rep. All other reps construct up to this point as fibers were recruited in sequence, and deeper inroads were made into starting strength levels through ever-increasing intensity.

It is not until that last, most uncomfortable repetition where the growth occurs. Bring an exercise set to this point and you can rest easy knowing that you have done enough to stimulate growth.

Do not apprehensive this entire book is not centered around fourth year college science but at the same time I want to make sure everyone recognizes exactly how our bodies are working. I did not break this book down in terms of a easy reading level because it takes too many words and most of this paraphernalia should be relatively common to most of you.

The anaerobic window mostly has an incorrect interpretation by that I mean people say that very high repetition ranges can stimulate as much growth because if you fail at rep 30, you have still progressed through the sequential recruitment. It is well agreed upon in the fitness world that sets lasting between 60-90 seconds or less will produce more in the way of anaerobic adaptations than aerobic ones. Our ability to recover from mechanical work is not unlimited, sets lasting more than one and a half minutes will split adaptations between both the aerobic and anaerobic systems. While there is nothing magical about a certain repetition number, a good repetition range and tempo should have you ending a set around the 1 minute mark. Therefore training systems that advocate very high rep ranges, or even the super slow movements, are not optimal for those highlighting muscular growth.

A question I often get from my clients is, "How do I know when I've reached failure?" When you think you may have reached failure, try another rep. If you achieve that rep, try another one and so on. Basically, a set does not end when you decide, it ends when your muscle fails. If you find that you can knock out 3 or 4 more repetitions every time you use this method, you are using weights that are too light. Often when people complain that they cannot reach failure, it is simply a case of submaximal loads. So increase the weight, there is nothing mysterious about failure, you will know it when you hit it.

Training not to failure can lead to what is called fake progression. If you use a weight that represents only 75% of a 10 repetition weight and lift a 10-rep set, you could progress for many months by increasing by a repetition here, an incremental weight increase there, and so on. Your numbers would be going consistently up but you would not be progressing in actuality because, in a few months' time you would finally reach the point where you lift 10 reps to failure with the weight you actually could have used way back at the start. This fake progression ensured that you never pressed through the upper parameters of your strength potential. As far as your body growing you would not actually be growing since you never forced any adaptation when you trained within your existing strength levels and never made any demand from your body to increase the size of the muscle fibers.

Training with the requisite intensity to trigger growth does involve a longer recovery period and this can confuse some people. Those bodybuilders who train the same body part 3 times a week will fall into this category.

By the time they perform their second workout of the week and are hitting the same muscle groups, they have not even recovered let alone overcompensated. Oftentimes, they will not be able to even repeat their previous performance let alone beat it. This than has a mental effect and a disappointing one which sometimes causes a person to go back to his old system, swearing never to train to failure again.

This extended recovery is for a very good reason though. Those powerful, type 2B fibers we want to hit, also take the longest to recuperate and overcompensate. The fact that you have pressed the growth control button and need that longer recovery time should put the over apprehensive bodybuilders mind at ease when he or she feels they are not training enough.

2 INTENSITY

Now that we have taken it to the next notch your method of training has changed and with that so has your intensity level. From now on you will not train to failure but past failure. It is virtually impossible to do this without a coach or a trainer or a workout partner. It just does not make sense. It is hard enough to train to failure but impossible to train past failure. Your muscles must be forced to train past failure. For a novice this method is a sure way to get you an ambulance ride to the hospital but by now you should have your form down. Doing this is going to trigger your bodies growth mechanism if you do not take it to this point there is very insignificant if any muscular growth being stimulated. You must also recall that the weight you are comfortable doing all the time for three sets will not help you with this program. You have to lift heavy, there is no two ways about it. Let us take an example; if you customarily do a set and max out at ten repetitions, if you were to stop at eight what would you accomplish? Nothing to stimulate your size and strength because you did not thrust yourself far enough or past your boundaries. It is when and only when you take your body past the point of failure, when your body feels like a rubber band, you cannot breathe, perspiration is dripping down your face and you feel like your veins are going to detonate that you know you have crossed that threshold.

Do not think there is not a mindset behind this because there is and if you have not mentally prepared yourself for this than it is not going to transpire. You must live, eat and breathe that this is what you want twenty four hours seven days a week. Go to sleep at night with zilch but training on your mind and when you awake in the morning it should be the first thing that grabs your attention. As you enter that gym all you should be focused on is pain and growth.

Any beginner or intermediate program will tell you to stop before failure because of the risk of injury but you will not have the sufficient stimulation to achieve maximum muscle growth if you do. Another guaranteed way to fail is any program that has you lifting the same weight in every set and taking that to failure. It is a good way to get a so called cut look but if you are reading this you want size and bulk and I am going to give that to you. We can get into the cutting stage at a later point of time.

I have been a strength training and conditioning , life coach and personal trainer for sixteen years and often hear my clients say I have seen amazing strength increases on this program. The only way you can certainly and accurately say that is if you had a genuine strength increase. You will be able to lift the same weight for more repetitions to failure than you did in your last workout or lift a heavier weight for the same or more repetitions. Will those other programs work? Yes, and they will keep you strong but will they build incredible mass? No! The reason why is because you are still training within your existing strength intensities.

Let me clarify this so you waste no more time trying techniques that do not work. If you go to the gym the next time and perform the same exercise for those ten repetitions but with a heavier weight and succeed you still have not progressed. The reason there was no progression is because you could have lifted the same weight in your previous workout. This can go on for weeks and months until finally one day you reach that point of failure.

Why would you want to waste that much time in getting yourself the bulk you want and deserve to have. I want you to start developing from day one and repetition number one with each and every set that you execute.

All of your advancements need to be tangible and by tangible I mean real strength. Look at this example if I was to see you today and tell you currently I curled twenty five pounds and every week I see you and I add one pound to that. In maybe two years you may see some progression but I would still be the same size. If you want to wait that long put the book down now because that is not what I am going to teach you.

This is how intensity breaks down, do you recollect the old pyramid training and so on? Forget about it. Every workout you are going to perform is going to start at the maximum. You are going to select a weight that is going to force you to have muscular failure within a given repetition range. Reflect on it this way, if you were to do ten sets and the last set was the only one that mandated you to failure, why did you waste your time on the other nine sets?

3 VOLUME

Now that we have established that a you are going to be performing a high intensity workout and that having high intense tension is a stipulation to stimulate growth we need to focus on the volume and sets.

Let us for a minute regress back to the old theories of more is better, it would make psychological sense to believe that but scientifically speaking it is actually been proven to be counterproductive.

One set is essentially just as effective as two to four sets per body part when trying to increase muscle size and strength after a ten week overall body training program.

The originator of the high intensity and low volume approach was essentially Arthur Jones, before his passing he actually said that bodybuilders who were interested in improving their muscular proportions and stamina should perform one set of each exercise to muscular failure. All of Arthur Jones advice has in the past been reviewed by the American College of Sports Medicine and found to be reinforced.

What this means to you is that additional growth stimulation will be transported to the muscles with supplementary high intensity sets but we also must keep in mind that there is a boundary to the amount of growth that can be stimulated in any single workout.

If you were to surpass the set and limit, the recovery period will become longer and once again we go back to the stage of being delayed. The term known as overtraining comes back into the realm of reality, a word no one wants to ever hear.

So what we need to do is add the third component in the next chapter that we added to the triangle called frequency to make sure we maximize our muscles with a precise, effective and efficient workout while ensuring we never over train or under train our bodies.

4 FREQUENCY

We can dissect frequency in two ways the first is we can stimulate the growth in each body part with just one set to failure and attack that body part multiple times per week in a full body routine or we can elect to stimulate growth in each body part with multiple sets but only hit each body part once a week in a five day split.

Here comes the million dollar question, why is it we cannot perform multiple sets per body part and still be able to hit that body part three times in a seven day period? The answer is; the more volume that you engage your body in, the more sets you do, and the longer your body will need to recover and grow.

Training your same body part over again before it has had a chance to adapt, will not allow that muscle to grow. This goes back to the basic fundamentals of why circuit training did not work because when we are working out we are breaking down muscle not building muscle. In order for our muscles to get bigger and grow they need rest. The same applies here.

Another way to describe this would be overcompensation. This would simply mean the body pulling back additional muscle than was there before the workout initiated and you do not and will not grow unless your body has had the time to recover.

If you were to complete too many sets what is going to materialize is you are going guarantee that by the time you are ready to work out that same body part again, that body part will not be ready to be worked out again resulting yet once more in overtraining.

Without getting too technical but still going back to what I had learned in college sufficient rest and recovery is needed between stress or training sessions this must take place in order for adaptation to occur. Adaptation will only occur during the inter training recovery periods and that any adaptation can return to a genetically determined previous training state if that stress is not properly maintained or developed properly.

This simply means for that in order to get the best results and to maximize muscle growth, we have to find your inner training point where you have achieved the maximum growth possible but before we begin to weaken again. That length of time is our goal.

We are going to achieve this with two cycles that you are going to rotate between. The first is going to be a five day split where you will work each body part once a week with multiple sets from Monday until Friday and the second is going to be a three day full body routine where you will work your whole body in one workout with one set until failure. It is in a way circuit training but with the proper techniques in place.

While one set taken to failure will stimulate growth, we now also know that by training in such a fashion that the typical person is recovered and has overcompensated in thirty six to forty eight hours and a three day a week routine will without a doubt work well.

If we are able to stimulate more muscle growth we could than take a longer lay off between training sessions which I know becomes an issue for many of you. We will however need to do this to allow for a full recovery. With a five day split which is a supported result driven plan you are going to get the maximum growth when you hit a body part to failure with numerous sets to failure.

You train for ten weeks with a five day split workout only working one to two body parts per session Monday through Friday and then you are going to take a full week off for a full system reclamation.

After your week off you are than going to start another ten week program where your training cycle will be a three day full body routine and again after that take a week off and its back to the five day split.

This ensures you do not hit the plateau state as well as you do not get bored.

Let me quickly touch on over compensating because the size of a muscle is directly proportional to its strength, if you are stronger on your next workout than you have over compensated. That being said if you complete more repetitions on the same exercise during your next workout you can be confident you have overcompensated.

In the past I conducted a private experiment with one of my clients and here was what I concluded.

It took four days to fully recover from just a single arm workout . I did this by taking my client beyond their normal state of failure and far beyond their intensity level that they ever experienced before. Therefore their recovery time was longer than it had ever been. Here is what makes it even more interesting, my client gained almost three quarter of an inch on their arms and that was the only exercise they performed for the rest of the week.

5 OVERLOADING

You now have the the six fundamentals behind us now, the three you already knew about and the three new ones I introduced to you. If you remember anything by reading this book it needs to be this chapter without it the rest has done nothing for you.

We spoke temporarily about overloading in the fundamental chapter so let us take a moment and recap. We now know that there is a point where our body must be set for our growth mechanisms to be properly triggered and that before we hit that point nothing at all is going to happen or at least no muscular growth will be stimulated which we began to call overloading the muscle.

Now what we want to accomplish is to overload the muscle. This just means that you cannot hang onto hitting the same weight for the same quantity of repetitions from workout to work out and anticipate to see the results you want.

Take something as simple as a barbell preacher curl, if you completed seven repetitions at eighty pounds this week to failure well the next time you have two choices; either you need to aim for eight repetitions or increase the weight to ninety pounds from repetition one. If you are honestly have problems getting to eight repetitions you should lower the weight a bit and go a little lighter (which is why I used it for an example).

Here is such a myth that we need to clear up, do not be tempted to quickly increase the weight by too much when you have achieved hitting twelve repetitions. This is such a downfall to many bodybuilders and is another reason behind plateauing. You need to increase the weights marginally to keep ensuring ongoing gains. Increasing your weight in the smallest increments possible is a sure fire win situation.

Whenever you perform more than one set of any exercise you are more than likely going to have to decrease the weight if you do successive sets. An example being, if you were to do nine reps at 100 pounds on your first set it is questionable you will get nine the second set. It is better to lift a bit lighter on the second and third set and so on. You would most likely refer to this as drop sets. Drop sets are a huge part of my program.

Imagine applying force to a pushbutton with your finger. Without a certain extent of pressure the button would not engage. However, once a very precise amount of pressure is applied, the button engages and triggers the electrical current that illuminates a light bulb. As far as kindling muscular hypertrophy, this precise amount of pressure is where the term overload is derived.

If you were to ask any personal trainer in the ecosphere of fitness and bodybuilding they would tell you the word overload simply means that the stress must be above the typical or customary level in order to get a succeeding transformation. If you apply that to weight lifting what we are saying is that the weight must be above a certain threshold or the adaptation will not occur. When we cross that brink we have than overloaded a muscle. Overloading is therefore required for producing muscle growth.

You really need to know how to overload that muscle. There are different methods to overload a muscle dependent on your objective. Some of these however are not pertinent or optimal when growth is your goal. They are however, increasing intensity, changing duration, changing the type or mode of the exercise and lastly changing the frequency of exercise.

I struggle that overloading a muscle when optimizing for growth is a matter of increasing reps and or load over time and increasing the intensity.

Changing the frequency is also significant and this feeds into my philosophy on what I have called intense overload.

The larger muscles are means they also have more of a metabolic appetite than smaller ones. Your body needs longer to recuperate and grow as you get bigger. As a bodybuilder you will notice that the more advanced you become and the more years you work out it appears like progress and growth takes longer to transpire. This means that in order to make continual gains you need a longer lay off period between workouts.

The gym is an addiction just like a drug so that being said we see the very opposite in the real world. All of us so called muscle heads that have been training for years head to the gym more and more often to force out new gains. Some of us, and myself not excluded even go twice a day rationalizing with ourselves that is a necessity because of our advanced rank. While I was employed at one health spa, I had to wear suit pants and a button down dress shirt and during work hours found myself working out so often that when it came time to work out I was so sore and exhausted. Reason being because if I added up the hours I worked out during the day it probably worked out to six hours. Through my own mistakes and more education here is what I learned, recovery takes longer for larger muscles, not shorter, so the logic is wrong. Apply the precise pressure, depress that button and illuminate that light bulb, then rest and allow the alteration to transpire.

There is a scientific understanding to the nature of increasing your muscle mass. Recite it and memorize it if you can! The following sentence may be the most important one you ever read in terms of gaining intelligence as well as a healthy and forever growing body.

"Sufficient rest or recovery between stresses, or training sessions, must be allowed for adaptation to occur. Adaptation will only occur during the inter-training recovery periods."

With that being said adaptation will only transpire during inter training recovery periods. If you bring the enticement back to the muscle before it has had satisfactory time to generate the adaptation, you will slow down any gain you were about to have. If larger muscles take longer to recover than the inter training periods must become longer to ensure that the muscles continue to grow. Overtraining is therefore one of the main reasons why intermediate and advanced bodybuilders make little or no progress.

6 INTENSE VOLUME

We just got finished discussing the five day split and if you paid attention you recognize you will perform a high volume of work. That is not to say you will be undertaking thirty sets per body part or that you will condense the intensity of the exertion you put forth. You are going to perform from five to nine sets per each body part and you will train to failure on each and every single set.

Here is how your weekly workout will look:

Monday – Shoulders and Traps

Tuesday - Legs

Wednesday – Chest and Abdominals

Thursday –Back and Biceps

Friday – Triceps

I want you to stick to the above plan as much as possible and the purpose why is to keep a forty eight hour time duration between shoulders and chest and triceps. When you work one of these muscles you are operating the other one or both. For the best possible recovery and maximum growth it is sensible to leave that forty eight hours between those body parts. You must also keep in mind that between legs and back workouts you want to do the same. You cannot squat without involving your back and you cannot deadlift without involving your legs.

You are always going to train to positive failure on each and every set and make sure you select a weight that will force you to reach failure amongst eight and twelve repetitions on every set.

Now this means you will have to use the drop set technique which means lowering the weight on successive sets of the same exercise. Great example if you get out nine repetitions completed on your first set of preacher curls at sixty five pounds, on your second set you will use fifty five to sixty pounds to ensure that you reach failure between eight and twelve repetitions. The tempo is raise for one to two seconds and then lower for two seconds.

You are going to want to allow some controlled loose form to kick in at the end of the set where and when it is practical and safe to do so. A good example are preacher curls, dumbbell lifts or barbell lifts. Deadlifts are a very poor example due to the hazard involved and because we all need proper form with deadlifts.

Use a rest pattern that stays consistent throughout all of your workouts and your cycle. When you take the same amount of rest between sets this will accurately form proper muscle progression.

Monday

When working shoulders and trapezoids start off by executing dumbbell lateral raises to failure and then quickly move to a set of overhead presses with no rest. The lateral raise will work the whole shoulder but seats most of the emphasis on the lateral deltoid which is the side. The overhead press on the other hand will work all three of the heads the anterior which is the front the lateral being the side and the posterior being the back.

The lateral head will be solely accountable for reaching positive failure on the lateral raises, the other two heads are not going to reach that punishing point of failure. Once we include more muscles into the compound overhead press we than push the lateral head beyond the point of positive failure and begin to stimulate the growth within that head.

The reason that I plan it out that way is because it is very easy to over train the anterior and posterior deltoids. You must keep in mind that the anterior deltoid is significantly involved in all chest exercises and the same applies to the posterior head in back movements as well as in some triceps movements. That all being said is why it is imperative to stimulate all three of the heads without overtraining which is also why you will need to do a pre exhaust set.

It is imperative to perform overhead presses while seated at a smith machine and this is because the muscle fibers of the shoulders will be so heated up and burning that it will be extremely difficult to maintain a proper balance while trying to perform these movements when using free weights.

You can use a variety of different trap bar shrugs, dumbbell or even e-z bar upright rows if you do not prefer doing cable shrugs.

Tuesday

Although squats and leg presses are awesome exercises please do not omit leg curls and leg extensions.

By doing this you are performing what I am sure you are aware are called isolation exercises which will place a maximum amount of demand and strain on your quadriceps and hamstrings. This is accomplished when the muscles are fully contracted and also called the peak contraction point. At this point all of the muscle fibers have become involved due to the range of motion.

A respectable leg day workout is going to consist of barbell squats, leg presses, leg extensions, leg curls and of course let us not forget calf raises. If you want to torture yourself a bit more at the end feel free to add some good ole wall sits.

Wednesday

My chest routines include the following the barbell bench press, pectoral deck with chest day I include abdominals so weighted sit ups as well as hanging leg raises.

I include the pectoral deck because by utilizing that machine your pectorals are fully contracted which is going to place a great amount of resistance on them. Once you have accomplished reaching muscular failure with the pectoral deck than transform over to using the compound movement and exercise called the barbell bench press which will of course involve other muscle groups including the shoulders and the triceps which is going to take your pectorals way past the point of positive failure.

Many individuals have the false conviction that to build abdominal muscles special machines and unusual exercises are required, well they are not. The ones I cited above are the ones I recommend because they place a multitude of stress on the abdominals at the peak contraction point. Any exercise that you can find that can do that is a great exercise. Now do not get me wrong many gyms have dedicated abdominal stations that are excellent do go ahead and take advantage of them to. Remember when you become strong enough or if you already are use additional weight to keep your legs straight and perform alternate reverse crunches.

Thursday

Thursdays are going to be our back and biceps day and will consist of deadlifts, barbell rows, decline cable pullovers, cable preacher curls and barbell curls. Please recall using optimized form works the best when performing bent over barbell rows, also if you have access to a pullover machine take advantage of it and use it.

Take yourself a five minute rest between moving from your back and blasting your biceps. You are going to notice another preliminary fatigue set that will bridge between the cable preacher curl and the barbell curl.

After you accomplish your third set to failure of cable curls, transfer immediately to the barbell curls without any rest period. Your biceps will be on fire at this point. After the preliminary fatigue calms down take a two minute break as typical and then perform two further sets of barbell curls.

Friday

Friday is triceps day and solitary triceps day, you will be performing French curls as well as triceps pushdowns. Although it does not seem like very much, after the four days of the penetrating workouts you had the previous days your body is going to be appreciating this day.

I myself certainly seem to enjoy the French curl and especially lowering the bar to your forehead really limits how much you can overload the stress you can place on your triceps. Ensure to allow some rotation at your shoulder joints by lowering the bar behind your head so you can really stimulate your triceps. Just do six straight sets. Three sets of French curls and three of the triceps pushdowns.

If you feel the necessity or have the additional energy on this day you can include a forearm exercise but more than likely your forearms will be sore from the weeks workout. If for some reason they are not than go ahead and include a set or two. Barbell wrist curls and dumbbell wrist curls are my preference.

7 BLAST CYCLE

So far we have discussed the ten week volume cycle than we take a week off after that let us move right into this cycle. Here is where you are going to work your whole body in one intense growth inspiring workout. You will be performing a solitary set per exercise and rest only about two to three minutes between the sets.

The rhythm you will be using is the three one three which broken down is lifting for a period of three seconds and then hold at the peak contraction point for a period of one second and then lower the weight for three seconds. There is not really any enhancement behind this rhythm but it does help the slow twitch muscles as well as hitting that negative repetition.

You will notice by using this type of tempo you are going to select a weight that forces failure within seven to ten repetitions excluding deadlifts which are five to eight repetitions.

The exact exercises I listed are important I have carefully researched them through the years and they have proven to be extremely effective in growth stimulation.

You will perform two massive phase workouts consisting of both isolation as well as compound exercises but you will mostly be doing isolation exercises. These exercises will be implemented on Monday and Wednesday

You are than going to follow that on Friday with a transitory third workout that will not be encompassing any isolation exercises. Without overstressing my point it does help with systemic recovery and will help to overcome plateaus and also hits those minor stabilizer muscles that we do not hit as effectively when we do isolation exercises.

The core of building muscle and understanding the true way it works it something you truly need to comprehend. In order to yield muscle growth you need to recruit as many muscle fibers as possible to stimulate that growth.

The best exercise for any body part is one that will work in conjunction with the function of that muscle. I know that may sound a bit confusing but it is really not. Your goal is to move your muscle into a position of maximum retrenchment or what they call a peak contraction point at this and only at this position will the most muscle fibers be engaged. The exercise at the same time must also encompass using maximum resistance while in this contracted point. This needs to be done in order to ensure that proper stimulation and muscle growth within the fibers is actually occurring.

There are so many programs out there and most of them work for the novice or individual who casually uses the gym once in a while. If you are reading this book you are more serious than that and need to concentrate on both isolation as well as compound exercises. At this stage isolation is going to give you some of your best and most effective results. Let me give you a great example: Let us take our biceps the primary function of the bicep muscle is to move the forearm towards the shoulder (elbow flexion). The secondary function of the bicep is supination of the forearm. That being said any movement of the bicep requires you to have the hands fully supinated with your palms turned up facing the ceiling and then moving your forearm up to meet your upper arm at this position you have just achieved maximum growth stimulation.

Let me help you put this puzzle together, I know it seems like a great deal of information packed into a chapter but I did not want to bore a person that already knows the basics with a bunch of basic information in other words no beating around the bush straight to the point.

I need to ensure that you are using enough resistance on the intended muscle when it is in its position of maximum contraction.

There is no doubt in my mind you have performed at slightest one set of standing barbell or dumbbell curls in your life. You should have noticed that the resistance falls off right after the mid-point of this exercise. All that means is that you were not at your maximum potential point and there was less than the optimal amount of resistance on your bicep.

I would strongly suggest trying to use the cable preacher curl machine as an alternate to the barbell or dumbbell preacher call. It is a very effective exercise and there is always even distribution of resistance throughout the range of motion. This exercise is going to ensure you work the bicep the correct way, the resistance will be greater and will cause the stimulated growth you are looking to achieve.

8 BLAST PHASE MONDAY, WEDNESDAY, FRIDAY

Remember Monday and Wednesday as well as Friday. So on Monday as well as Wednesday you will perform seven to ten reps of each exercise.

Legs
Squats

Laterals
Pull downs

Shoulders
Lateral Raise
Overhead Press

Biceps
Cable Preacher Curl

Triceps
Pushdowns

Chest
Pectoral Deck

Traps
Cable Shrugs

Calves
Calf Raises

Wrists
Dumbbell Wrist Curl

Abs
Decline Sit Up

There are three compound movements in the above workout. You have squats, pull downs and overhead presses. I want no pausing at any range of motion when you are doing your squats and overhead presses because there really is no point of hard contraction. Stick to the three, one, three rule when lowering the weight and then simply push the weight up under control for the positive. Pull downs are accomplished in the same manner as the isolation exercises in the three one three fashion

From the commencement of this book we are going to stimulate growth by taking set number one to failure and we are only going to do one of each of the exercises above to failure. Mentally this is going to be the toughest part.

Ensure you have picked a weight for yourself that will force failure between the seventh and the tenth repetition

When doing these sets I want you to take a good two to three minute rest between those sets and certainly concentrate when you are taking that rest period on what the next exercise is so you can mentally prepare yourself for that next set.

Just as we discussed with the other cycle the third set is going to become a preliminary fatigue on your shoulders and there will be no rest.

Your triceps and your pectorals will habitually conflict with each other but they are not going to with this program. Most of us would like to use the bench press to stimulate our chest growth the problem here is that the movement is also involving the triceps to such a large degree. Both the pushdowns and pectoral deck are both isolation movements that will cause no such conflict.

Most gyms these days and notice I said most gyms, have a floor pulley system to use for cable shrugs if not use a barbell or if your gym has a trap shrug bar use that.

I have carefully chosen these exact exercises. I also carefully arranged the order in which I want them to be performed. If you follow the order as well as the program to a tee you will be working your synergists and fixator muscles prior to working the agonist or prime mover.

FRIDAY

Back – Deadlifts 5 to 8 repetitions

Biceps and Laterals – palms up pull downs 7 to 10 repetitions

Triceps and shoulders and Chest – Dips 7 to 10 repetitions

Legs – Squats 7 to 10 repetitions

Try to remember that dissimilarity sessions are brief and compound only exercises.

When we try to challenge to recruit the maximum number of fibers for a given muscle we are demanding that it be worked according to its function. By incorporating this we are placing meaningful resistance in its maximum contracted position. For the most part doing this is going to require the use of isolation exercises.
That is not however to say that by us favoring isolation exercises we are not drawing back or discounting a number of small muscles because we are. We only activate those other muscles when we do compound lifts. Now not only do these muscles contribute to full muscular development but they also help to control and prevent plateaus. If your stabilizer muscles are underdeveloped you will most likely plateau during certain lifts where they come into play.

Also keep in mind that these consolidation workouts will help with what is known as universal recovery.
The lower intensity and the lower volume will never make as large of an impact on your recovery ability.

This is very important just as with the point I stated above concerning compound movements in this phase there is no pausing with deadlifts, dips or leg presses. These muscles are never actually brought into a position of maximum contraction because it is physically impossible. Stick with a three second lowering of the weight but do not focus on rhythm on the positive, just simply push the weight up with control. Remember palms-up pull downs are accomplished in the same manner as the isolation exercises as the 3 to 1 to 3 tempo.

You once again will choose a weight that will cause failure between the seventh and tenth repetition except of deadlifts where you should be selecting a weight that forces failure between the fifth and eighth repetition.

Take a four minute rest between these sets. This workout is all about building overall strength and creating the new huge you as well as increasing the weight for all these heavy compound movements. If you want to achieve new goals and records taking that break will give your body the rest it needs to do it.

9 CARDIO

I already know I am opening a can of worms including cardio in this book but at the same time if I do not I am going to leave a cluster of unanswered questions. The philosophy I use for beginner and intermediate clients is the ten to fifteen minutes of cardio followed by thirty minutes of strength training and then followed by thirty minutes of cardio.

Now that you are in the advanced if not professional phase I am going to change it up a bit. Adding extra cardio sessions on top of your weight training is comparable to driving your car with one foot on the accelerator and the other depressing the clutch. While you may be moving forward, you are heading to your destination at a slower rate than you would if you would just take your foot off the clutch.

Let us look at the reasons individuals are adding cardio on top of their weight training:

First and foremost to burn calories and try to stay lean all year round while they build muscle concurrently and or to preserve or advance cardiovascular fitness while they bulk up. I want to be unblemished on my position from the inception here; there is no merit to either of these points. Let us now inspect these in greater detail.

First of all, cardio is suggested when fat loss is of significance. It is said to be intelligent to split your bodybuilding lifestyle into periods of bulking and cutting, the question is, should you maintain cardio throughout your bulking cycle?

Many athletes and personal trainers will tell you that it is a good idea, others will tell you it is not. I agree with the latter group. If you want to maintain a lean physique while stimulating growth all year round, here's how to do it:

Eat a diet that provides no more than what you need for growth most of the time. Remember the 80/20 rule; if you do things right 80% of the time, you can afford to do them wrong 20% of the time.

Ideally, by governing your blood sugar you are releasing fat storing insulin by living a low medium glycemic load lifestyle. This is the diet you need. Doing things wrong 20% of the time will lead to gradual fat-gain. Counter this with infrequent mini-cuts.

This is a much better way of staying lean year-round.

Cardio is not as effective as you might think. When you journey onto a treadmill, it will ask you to input your weight, this is for a specific reason: it is calculating your resting metabolic rate (RMR). This is vital to recognize since when you have finished your session and see 400 calories burned on the screen, this is 400 total calories including the calories you would have burned just lying on the sofa. If your RMR was 1900 and you consumed an hour burning that 400 calories, you really burned about an extra 320 calories, not 400. Eat an typical chocolate bar and you have undone an hour's work in 5 minutes.

We did not evolve to burn calories effortlessly. If we did, we probably would not be here right now. Our ancestors would have perished of starvation during long periods without food because hunting would have expended mega calories. The fact that the body does not burn calories very easily was a big plus for our ancestors but a discomfort for modern man. We live in a society of food surplus where high calorie snacks are never far away. For evolutionary reasons, our body will want to store this excess energy as fat for times of food scarcity that never actually come.

We are always somewhere between the polar ends of anabolism and catabolism. From the perspective of the guy who wants to build muscle and be in anabolism as much as possible all that running tips the scales more in favor of catabolism and must be seen as a negative.

Let us take a closer look at this anabolism and catabolism thing, To understand this, you first need to understand the way in which the body builds muscle. A bodybuilding workout does not build muscle, it just stimulates the body's own growth machinery into action. Once you have stimulated growth with a workout that represented a progression and was of sufficient intensity, a second process now begins: We call these processes recovery and growth.

Your body will not build a gram of new muscle until it fully recovers that which was lost in the workout. Only once the recovery process is finalized can your body then overcompensate. It is fairly simple logic that would dictate that anything that makes the recovery process longer is not good if your goal is to increase the total mass of muscle on your body.

The shorter the recovery, the quicker you get into your growth mode. Some may contemplate that only further weightlifting and especially working the same muscle group will eat into recovery but that is where another popular misconception lies. Any mechanical work of at least moderate intensity or higher, beyond that which is required to stimulate growth in muscle mass eats further and further into recovery and therefore prevents overcompensation, cardio is a bad idea from the perspective of the bodybuilder.

Any extra work, cardio or otherwise since it is all mechanical work, actually prevents building mass at the rate that would be conceivable if you would just rest and let the body do what it does all by itself.

Now, are you doing cardio for maximum improvements to your cardiovascular system? That is, do you want to be fit as well as muscular? If so, cardio is still a bad idea. It has been proven that just 6 minutes of high intensity exercise, 2 to 3 times a week, is very effective in improving aerobic fitness. Endurance was increased by almost 100%. This test was done against a group who participated in jogging, cycling, and aerobics and even though not in any structured manner their endurance did not improve at all.

The high intensity group however showed a significant increase in a chemical known as citrate synthase which is an enzyme that is indicative of the tissue's power to use oxygen. The group that achieved such improvements were using a 30-second sprint protocol. Remembering that this is simply mechanical work by the muscles, high intensity weight training will yield the same, if not even a better result. After some sets, like deadlifts to failure, I am more wiped than anything I could achieve with training on a bike or treadmill. It is not desirable to do both from the bodybuilder's point of view for reasons stated above and full recovery growth.

Now, could weight-lifting, an anaerobic activity, benefit the aerobic pathways more than cardio? I know this sounds counter intuitive but let us have a closer look. When we talk about improvements to the cardiovascular system, we are really taking about are metabolic adaptations within the cells that the cardiovascular system supports. It may seem surprising that it is actually during recovery from weight training or anaerobic activity that the aerobic system reaps benefits at least equal to, and often greater than, steady state cardio and aerobics. This will require a quick look at cell metabolism.

Anaerobic metabolism in the cytosol portion of the cell turns glucose into pyruvate.

Pyruvate is then moved into the mitochondria where it is aerobically metabolized to become thirty six molecules of adenosine triphosphate.

Glycolysis only produces two molecules of adenosine triphosphate but cycles much faster than the Krebs cycle/respiratory chain which produces 36 molecules of adenosine triphosphate.

When involved in high-intensity training, like lifting to failure, you turn the glycolytic cycle and produce pyruvate more rapidly than it can be used by the aerobic cycle.

As the additional pyruvate builds up it is converted to lactic acid, explaining why you feel the burn during your workouts.

It is only through this type of intense, anaerobic activity that you force the Krebs cycle aerobic to turn as quickly as possible to deal with the large ingestion of pyruvate into the mitochondria. Jogging, running, rowing are just not as effective for this.

While recovering from intense muscular contractions, the lactate that builds up is then transformed back into pyruvate which then has to be aerobically absorbed. This means that your aerobic system is stimulated while you rest and recover from lifting weights. The aerobic system works at its highest level when recovering from lactic acidosis. You are indeed getting much fitter by working with weights and recovering from the same.

You can now disregard all the comments you hear so many individuals who repeatedly accuse muscular guys of being unfit because they do not do cardio. Keep in mind that through progressive overload we are growing stronger all the time. Since the musculature is being served by the aerobic system, improvements in muscle strength and size will also result in upregulation of the aerobic system.

Aside from the above points about simply controlling caloric intake, intense weight training will mobilize warehoused fat by activating hormone sensitive lipase. Hormone sensitive lipase releases these fatty acids which are then transported to the muscles. Beta oxidation forms thirty five molecules of adenosine triphosphate from them. This is unique to emergency situations and high-intensity muscular work that calls into play our powerful type 2b muscle fibers which of course is an event that has been catered for you in my training.

Let me summarize it this way if you are doing cardio to burn calories just do not eat them in the first place. You are already keeping fit with weight training. The added aerobics is counterproductive when we understand the processes of inroading and overcompensation.

10 PROTEIN

Having enough protein in your diet is essential for building muscle. Knowing just how much is enough can be a little tricky for some people so I have decided to set the record straight in this book. Listening to the average person at the vitamin store who was flipping burgers last week or the guy trying to sell you a fitness membership at the local health spa all the way to your primary physician about how much protein you need in your diet is simply not going to cut it for the bodybuilder.

What type of people are primary physicians used to seeing? Normal average muscular people to overweight individuals, so when asked a question about protein and the bodybuilder do not be surprised if you get a dumbfounded look or expression. You need more than the average person protein wise simply because your muscle tissue is constantly being ripped.

The best method of calculating just how much protein is enough for a high protein diet is with the following formula.

Lean Mass Weight (Kg) x 2.75 = Daily Protein Requirement

By the way you simply divide pounds by 2.2 to get the equivalent in Kilograms. So 150 pounds is 68.18 Kg

You first need to know your total body weight and your body fat percentage. If you do not know your body fat percentage and you are at this stage of the bodybuilding game you have issues.

Take your body fat percentage. Multiply this percentage by your total body weight to determine the amount of fat you are carrying. Now simply subtract this from your total body weight to determine your lean mass weight.

Take this figure and multiply it 2.75 to give you your ideal protein intake per day in grams.
Example
A man weighs 150 pounds with 15% body fat.
150 / 2.2 = 68.18 Kg
15% x 68.18 = 10.23 Kg
68.18 – 10.23 = 57.95 Kg – Lean body mass in Kg
57.95 x 2.75 = 159.36
So, therefore our 150 pound, 15% body fat man should be shooting for 159 grams of protein in his daily diet.

ABOUT THE AUTHOR

Born in Astoria Queens, New York Tim Taylor has become one of the most world renowned personal trainers and author. His book publications include The Body Bible, The ABCs OF A LEAN SCUPTED BODY as well as his release of Breaking The Mold as well as ongoing and continuing works still in progression. Tim's goal is to be able to share his knowledge of the exercise and fitness world with people who are mostly taken down the wrong road with miss-informative articles dealing with exercise, health and fitness.

Tim is the owner of a successful personal training studio, conducts boot camps and gives health and fitness seminars worldwide on a regular basis. His publications and seminars are used for educational and teaching of both new and up and coming certified personal trainers as well as for experienced body builders and fitness models.

Tim prides himself on making his clients reach their fitness goals and states that is what keeps him motivated to continue training, writing and inspiring individuals.

Tim still takes on new clients that are serious and success driven and states that out of all the careers he could have chosen in life no other career could provide the same amount of satisfaction of knowing you have truly helped someone turn a dream into a reality.

www.ingramcontent.com/pod-product-compliance
Lightning Source LLC
Chambersburg PA
CBHW081801280526

45789CB00008B/2956